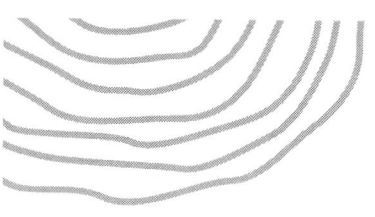

## Day 1

This morning I made myself pancakes:
Oats with banana, cinnamon, honey and milk
Dressed them with grapes, raspberries, blueberries
and blackberries – all the berries with glossy curves
remind me of what women's bodies do
–
burst with ink.

-Lisa de Jong

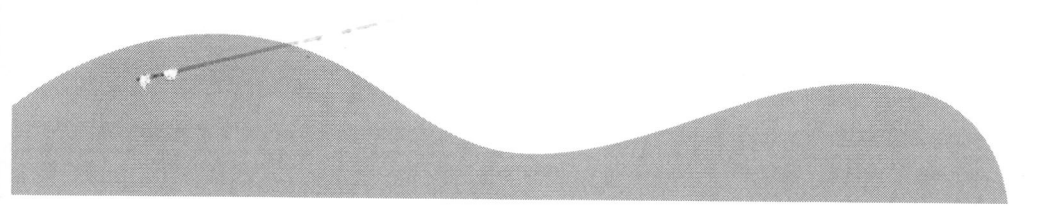

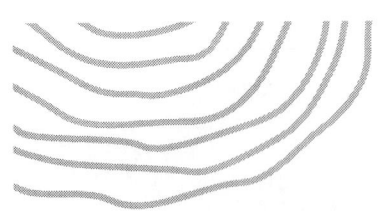

"So don't be frightened, dear friend, if a sadness confronts you larger than any you have ever known, casting its shadow over all you do. You must think that something is happening within you, and remember that life has not forgotten you; it holds you in its hand and will not let you fall. Why would you want to exclude from your life any uneasiness, any pain, any depression, since you don't know what work they are accomplishing within you?"

-Rainer Maria Rilke

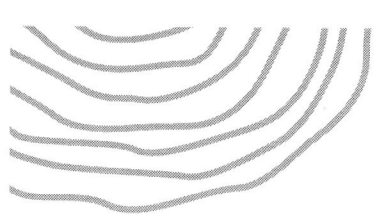

# Intention

My intention for this journal:

_____
_____
_____
_____
_____
_____
_____
_____
_____
_____
_____
_____
_____
_____
_____
_____
_____
_____
_____
_____
_____
_____
_____
_____
_____
_____
_____
_____

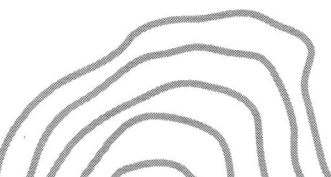

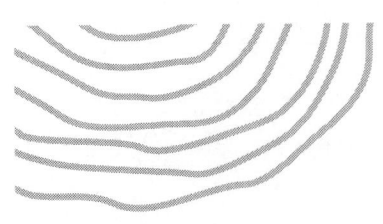

# Welcome

Welcome, and thank you for being curious about tracking your menstrual cycle!

The menstrual cycle is a hugely important part of a woman's health and has been a bit forgotten about in daily well-being. The cycle is linked to our endocrine system, our nervous system and our immune system, therefore, it can be hugely beneficial to explore it in more depth. Tracking the cycle will support you on your journey to wellness, any kind of recovery linked to menstrual health, a fertility journey, a journey through therapy, healing through trauma, grief and also during times of transition. Use this journal daily, perhaps placing it next to your bed so you can make a daily log. The notes taken can offer valuable information for your doctor, therapist and most importantly – yourself! This journal can also be used for anyone wanting to live in sync with their cycle for creativity, productivity and better understanding of the body.

If you experience irregularities in your cycle, tracking it can unveil hidden trends and bring awareness to the body on different days of the cycle – I would still encourage you to track. If you do not have a womb or if you are no longer menstruating, you can use this journal to track your experiences through the lunar (moon) cycle.

This journal is about developing a relationship with the menstrual cycle so that we, as women, and people with cycles, can feel fully connected in our bodies and therefore lead wholehearted lives.

# How to use this journal

This journal is specially designed to allow you to explore your menstrual cycle in more depth and intimacy than an app, however, it can be used alongside an app of course! The layout is such that all day 1s are together, all day 2s are together and so on, for 12 cycles. This lets you very easily and clearly identify trends in your own experience for each phase of the cycle and will bring your personal practice of Menstrual Cycle Awareness to a deep and practical level.

For example, you may log a headache or an argument with someone repeatedly on a particular day or phase of the cycle for a few months. Because the same day of each cycle is next to each other in the journal, trends will be easy to spot and will then give you an indication of what areas to address and prioritise in terms of health, relationships and life in general.

Each quadrant allows for a day of the menstrual cycle, beginning with day 1. Mark the date for your own records and take note of how you feel or anything that stands out in terms of your physical, emotional, mental and spiritual experience that day. For Fspiritual, this can be how connected you feel to yourself, others and the world or whatever spirituality means to you! Sometimes, just a few lines or even a word to capture the tone of the day is enough. Go with what feels right. What you write, how you record it and how much you write, will also reveal significant insights over time.

I suggest that you also make a note of any dreams that stand out and write something you're grateful for because gratitude brings positivity and healing to our minds.

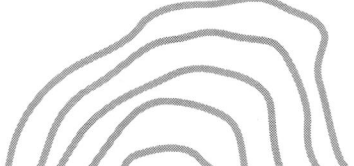

# How to use this journal

**Some areas to consider for each heading:**

- **Physical:** food cravings, appetite, cervical fluid, libido, exercise, joints, discomfort or ease, sleep quality, bowel movements, how the body feels in general.
- **Mental:** general thoughts, worries, attitude, mindset, the inner critic, comparisons, ideas, inspiration, motivation
- **Emotional:** any major feelings that come up or the general tone of the day
- **Spiritual:** how connected you feel to yourself, the spirit world, creativity or nature

**Here is an example:**

> Day 2, 30/3/17
>
> Physical: quite crampy, achy, weak and tired most of the day but not all bad. Cancelled some work and slept in the afternoon. My blood is nice and red today. It looks healthy. Hungry in the evening. Craving pizza and chips!
>
> Emotional: Did a meditation in the afternoon and felt really comfortable in the stillness - more than usual. Woke up feeling peaceful and loved after a nap!
>
> Mental: At poetry class in the evening, I felt more comfortable in myself and could access a vulnerability well. Trying not to be too hard on myself.
>
> Something I'm grateful for: The kind lady in the poetry class who is always friendly

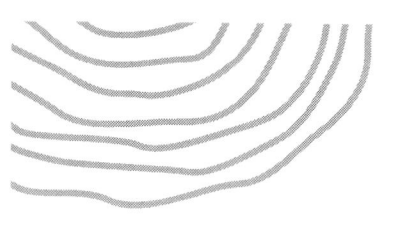

# What is Menstrual Cycle Awareness?

Menstrual Cycle Awareness (MCA) is a mindfulness practice that takes into account which day of the menstrual cycle we are on and how we feel and experience the world in relation to that day. Like all mindfulness practices, it is non-judgemental awareness of the day of the cycle and how we feel physically, mentally, emotionally and spiritually throughout that particular day.

Experiencing a menstrual cycle means that our hormones are doing different things every day. It's almost like having a different physiological make up on each day of the cycle and for that reason, it's both important and interesting to explore this part of the body as it is connected to all areas of health.

Practicing MCA brings mindfulness to a somatic and body-aware level and will therefore give us more insight into ourselves as physical beings in the world. Over time, we may identify trends, common challenges, strength and vulnerabilities at different times in the cycle. The journey of tracking the cycle in this way will allow for more self-compassion, understanding and clarity on how best to look after ourselves as cyclical beings.

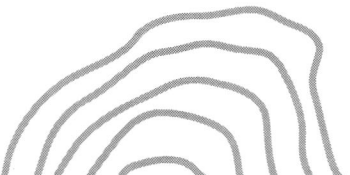

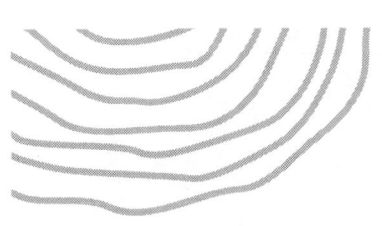

# The Inner Seasons

## INNER WINTER
### Follicular Phase

The first day of your period is the first day of blood flow, not including any spotting before. This is day 1 of your menstrual cycle. However, you may feel a huge drop in energy, or mood changes a day or two before day 1 of your cycle – which marks the transition to Inner Winter.

During this phase, all hormonal levels are low and oestrogen will pick up gradually over the next few days. You may experience menstrual cramps, headaches, other aches and pains and emotions. On an energetic level, your body is dropping into the darkness of Winter. This is one of the most important and significant phases of the menstrual cycle but it can also be the most difficult. You may need to take painkillers, sleep, drink plenty of fluids or anything else that nourishes your body during this time.

The self-care task for you at this point is to – surrender – where possible. Even if it's just to lie down and breathe for 15 minutes. For some women, it's taking a day off work. Whatever feels right for you. Do it! You deserve it as it's the body's optimal time for renewal restoration. The way you allow yourself to menstruate sets the tone for the rest of the cycle and as women, we have an in-built reminder to take down time. It's important you do in whatever way you can.

Once you've surrendered, you may experience feelings of restlessness or boredom. This is normal and perfectly ok! Many of us are not used to taking time off every month or, we may want to escape some kind of suffering.

Acknowledge and dignify your own experience to yourself and do what you can to be kind to yourself. My suggestion is to not rush out of your Winter cave too soon. Go gently. Otherwise we risk burnout during the ovulatory phase of the cycle.

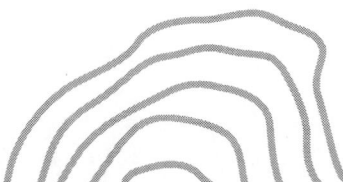

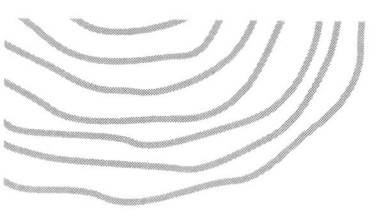

# The Inner Seasons

## INNER SPRING
### Follicular Phase

This phase typically happens from around days 6-11 and there can still be light bleeding at the start. Usually, you may feel a rise in energy and a lightness in your being which marks the onset of Spring. It's as if the outer lights of the world begin to slowly turn on. Gradually, our mental focus moves outward.

If you have moved slowly and gently out of Winter, this phase is all about fun, innocence and joy. Similar to the outer season of spring, your shoots are vulnerable still and need lots of gentleness. Think of spring lambs playing innocently in the field and the growth of new flowers like daffodils. This is a time to truly cherish yourself in whatever way you can.

Going for walks without an intention, playing with something creative with no particular goal in mind, lying in the bath and reading a nice book. Even, choosing "doing nothing" for some time and as my teacher, Alexandra Pope taught me – pissing away time – just because!

If, however, you have rushed out of your Winter cave or if you feel and follow the need to *do do do*, then this phase can become quite difficult leaving you feeling tired, depressed, depleted and with low emotional resilience. Do what you can to Cherish Yourself. Move tenderly.

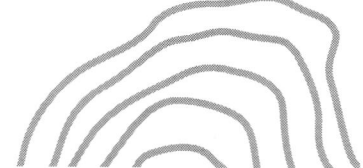

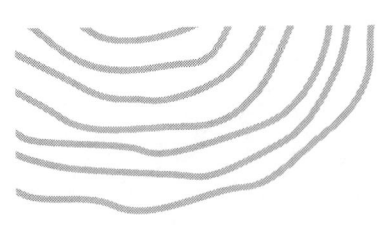

# The Inner Seasons

## INNER SUMMER
### Ovulation

The ovulatory phase of the cycle is typically from around days 12-19 and is the fertile phase, but again, this differs from woman to woman. Oestrogen is at its highest, which means your energy is peaking. The outer lights are fully switched on now.

During this phase, you may have noticeable physical changes such as increased vaginal discharge and some women can feel their ovulation happening on one side of the lower abdomen. This is called mittelschmerz and can sometimes be a bit uncomfortable or painful. Energetically speaking, you can feel super sexy, broody, very creative, sociable, confident, emotionally resilient and it's as if you are super woman. You can take care of lots of people and get all the jobs done – no problem.

Sometimes however, it can feel like life is great and it will never change. We forget during this phase that we are in a cycle and we can become a bit disillusioned by all our power and energy. Be careful with this. If we allow our Inner Summer to take over our agenda, we may face the consequences in the seasons to come. We can then feel regret in a couple of weeks with too many work and social commitments!

During Summer, the best way to look after your being is to declare or show yourself to the world. Go on that date, wear that outfit you've been shying away from, try that new lipstick, get stuck into that new creative project, do the work. Be your wonderful and loving self and relish every moment! Let yourself shine in the world!

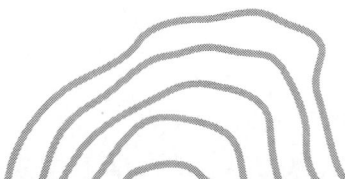

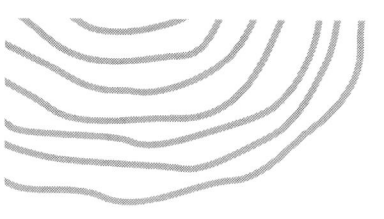

# The Inner Seasons

## IINNER AUTUMN – PRE MENSTRUATION
### Luteal Phase

During this phase, oestrogen beings to decline and progesterone is released and rises as a result of ovulation. This phase is typically from days 20-28. It is marked first by a calming after the height of inner summer, and then by a drop in energy with tiredness, an urge to complete tasks and perhaps mood changes such as irritability or general sensitivity. The outer lights of the world are turning off and the inner lights are turning on. It can be overwhelming to be in the busy world towards the end of this phase with the natural pull inward.

Socially, the premenstrual phase has been the subject of derogation for many years, calling women moody, snappy or grumpy. However, this is actually the no nonsense, truth speaking time of the cycle. We see things as they really are. This is a time to meet our inner critic, to complete projects, to speak up, to edit our work, to have that difficult conversation.

Similar to the outer season of autumn, we begin to let go of that which we no longer need. What is no longer serving us? How can we best prepare for the cave of Inner Winter? Many women suddenly feel a strong urge to clean and tidy or to organise something. This is a great time for finishing off loose ends, getting food and other things ready that will support our surrender during Winter.

It is important that during this phase we slow down energetically. We begin to say no to things and create space for ourselves. If you suffer in some way during this phase, getting creative can be a great remedy for that, as can movement such as dance or yoga.

If you find yourself mouthing off a lot during this phase, take heart, you are not alone! The task for you is to face yourself and to hold the tension. Feel those feelings of frustration, look at the role you've played, bring in some self-compassion and perhaps carry that something that has been bothering you through the next cycle to handle it more lovingly.
Letting yourself have a good cry can be hugely healing during this phase.

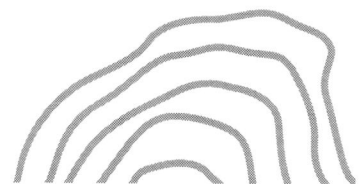

# Day 1

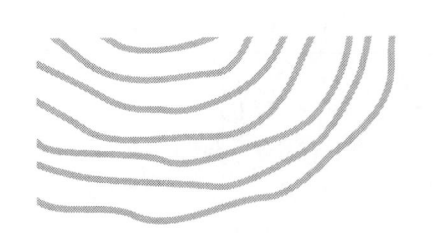

DATE

DATE

DATE

DATE

# Day 1

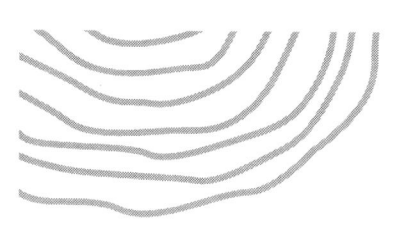

| DATE | DATE |
|---|---|
| | |

| DATE | DATE |
|---|---|
| | |

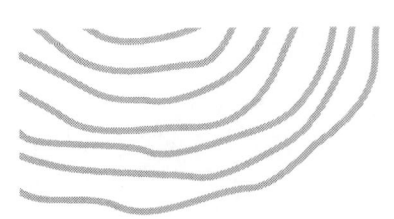

# Day 1

DATE

DATE

DATE

DATE

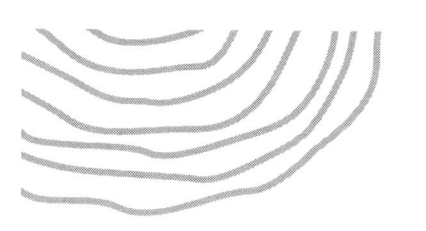

# Reflections

# Day 2

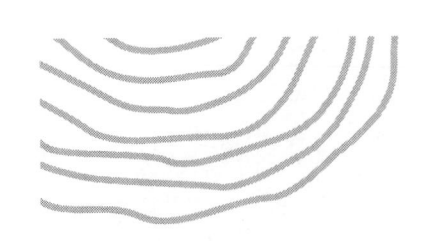

DATE

DATE

DATE

DATE

# Day 2

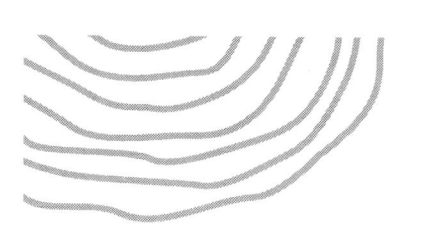

| DATE | DATE |
|---|---|

# Day 2

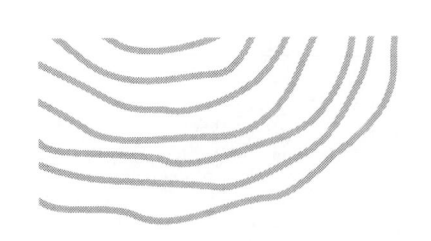

DATE

DATE

DATE

DATE

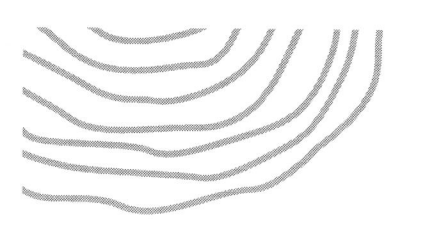

# Reflections

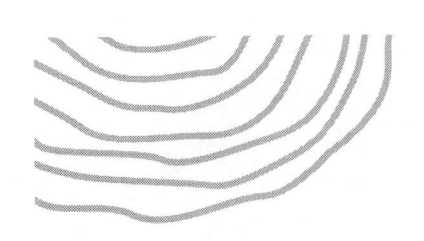

# Day 3

**DATE**

**DATE**

**DATE**

**DATE**

# Day 3

**DATE**

**DATE**

**DATE**

**DATE**

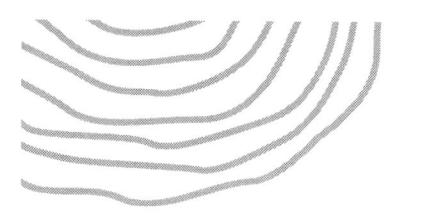

# Day 3

| DATE | DATE |
|---|---|

| DATE | DATE |

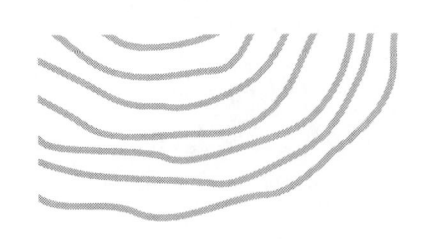

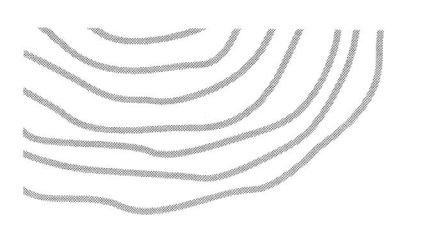

# Reflections

# Day 4

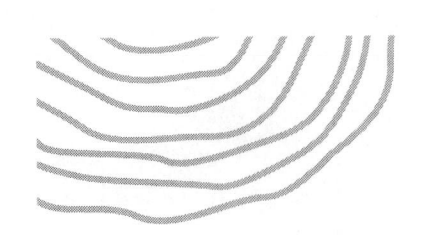

DATE

DATE

DATE

DATE

# Day 4

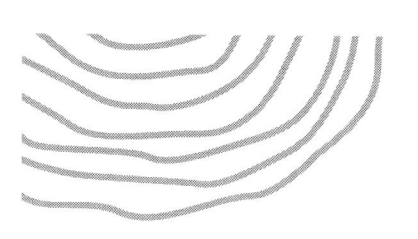

DATE

DATE

DATE

DATE

# Day 4

DATE

DATE

DATE

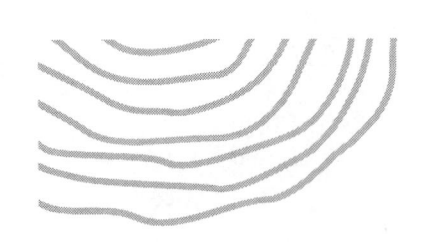

DATE

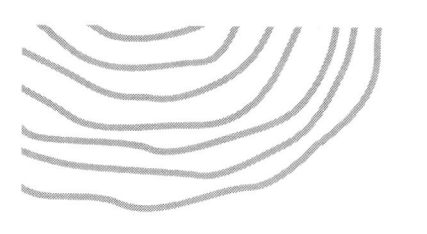

# Reflections

# Day 5

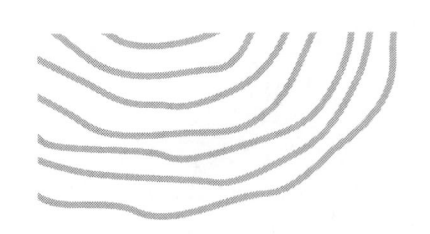

| DATE | DATE |
|---|---|
| | |

| DATE | DATE |
|---|---|
| | |

# Day 5

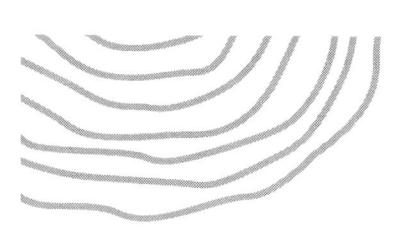

DATE

DATE

DATE

DATE

# Day 5

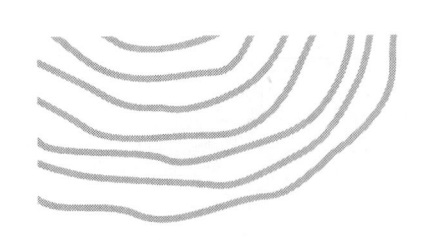

**DATE**

**DATE**

**DATE**

**DATE**

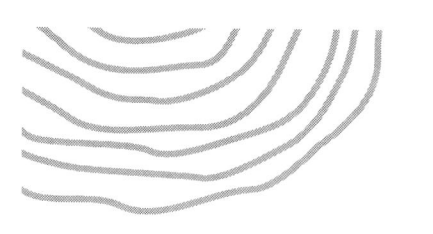

# Reflections

# Day 6

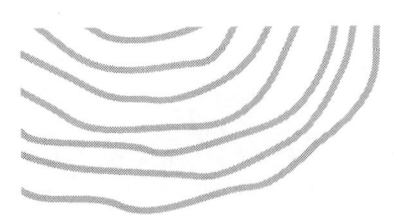

**DATE**

**DATE**

**DATE**

**DATE**

# Day 6

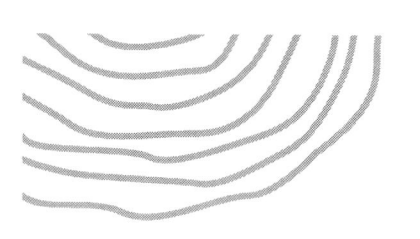

| DATE | | | | | DATE | | | |
|---|---|---|---|---|---|---|---|---|

# Day 6

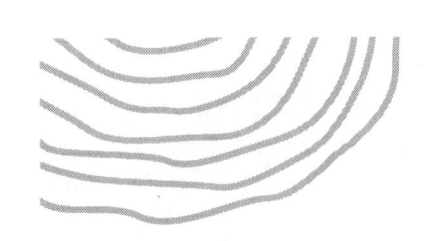

DATE

DATE

DATE

DATE

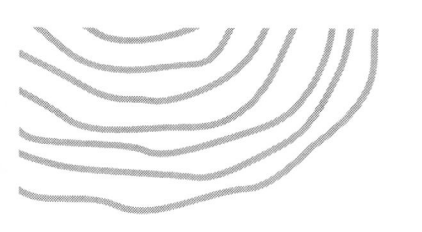

# Reflections

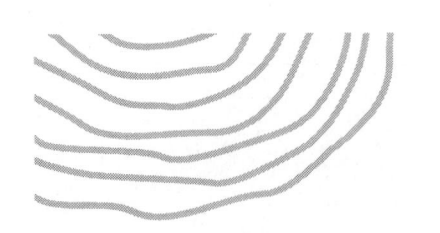

# Day 7

DATE

DATE

DATE

DATE

"If every tiny flower wanted to be a rose, spring would lose its loveliness."
~ St. Therese of Lisieux

# Day 7

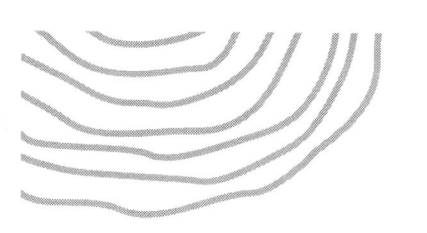

DATE

DATE

DATE

DATE

"I am not afraid... I was born to do this."
~ Joan of Arc

# Day 7

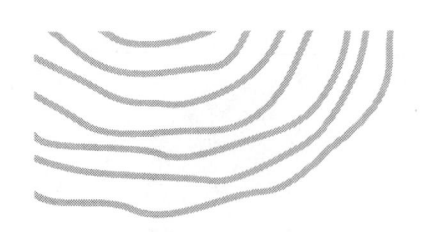

DATE

DATE

DATE

DATE

"If you desire faith, then you have faith enough."
~ Elizabeth Barrett Browning

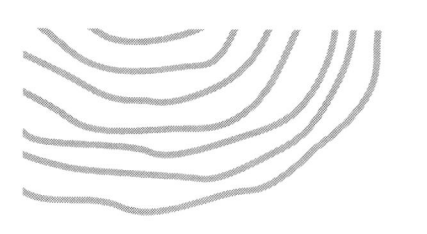

# Reflections

# Day 8

| DATE | | DATE | |
|---|---|---|---|

| DATE | | DATE | |
|---|---|---|---|

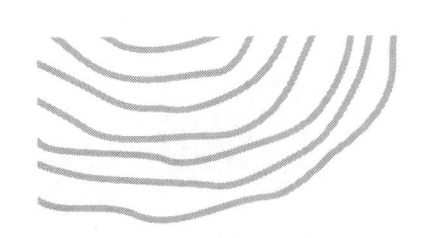

# Day 8

DATE

DATE

DATE

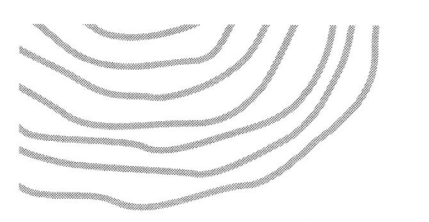

DATE

# Day 8

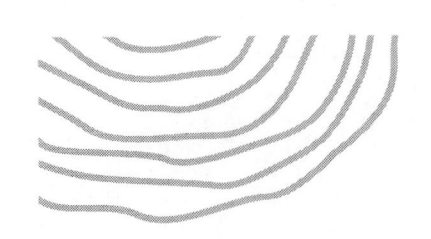

**DATE**

**DATE**

**DATE**

**DATE**

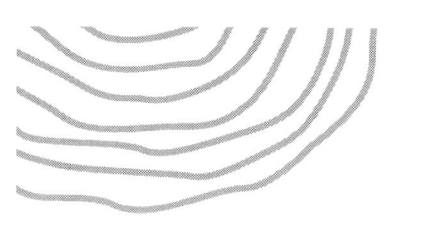

# Reflections

# Day 9

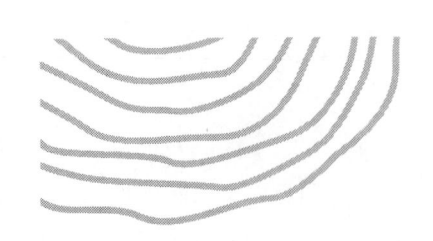

DATE

DATE

DATE

DATE

# Day 9

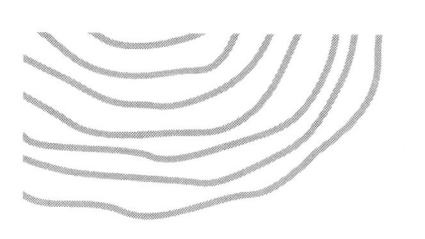

DATE

DATE

DATE

DATE

# Day 9

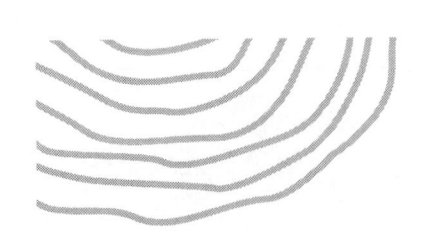

DATE

DATE

DATE

DATE

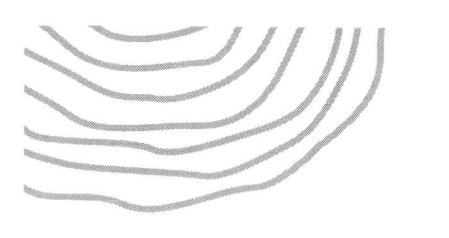

# Reflections

"Twenty years from now you will be more disappointed by the things that you didn't do than by the ones you did do. So throw off the bowlines. Sail away from the safe harbor. Catch the trade winds in your sails. Explore. Dream. Discover."
~ Mark Twain

# Day 10

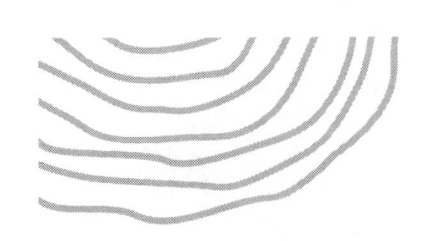

**DATE**

**DATE**

**DATE**

**DATE**

# Day 10

DATE

DATE

DATE

DATE

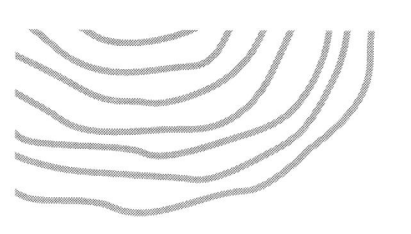

# Day 10

| DATE | | DATE | |
|---|---|---|---|

| DATE | | DATE | |
|---|---|---|---|

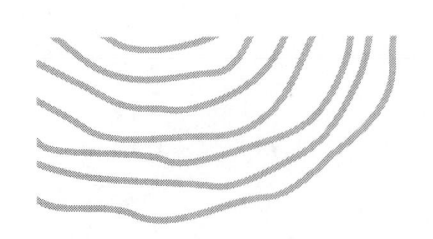

# Reflections

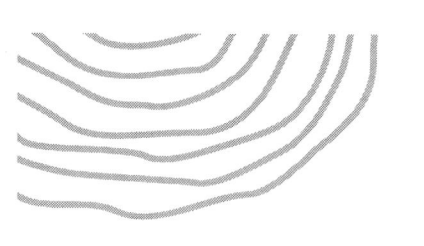

# Day 11

| DATE | DATE |
|---|---|
| | |

| DATE | DATE |
|---|---|
| | |

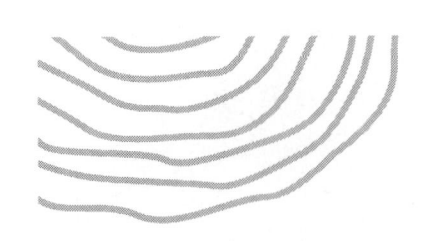

# Day 11

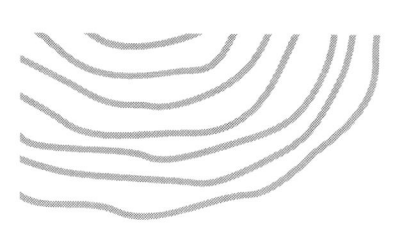

| DATE | | DATE | |
|---|---|---|---|

# Day 11

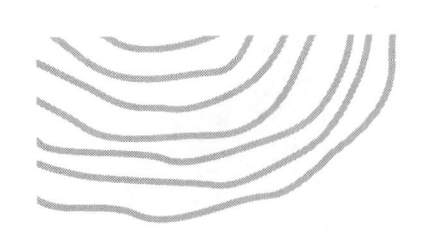

DATE

DATE

DATE

DATE

# Reflections

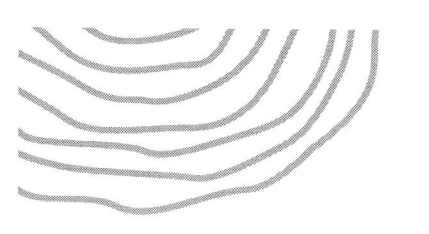

# Day 12

DATE

DATE

DATE

DATE

# Day 12

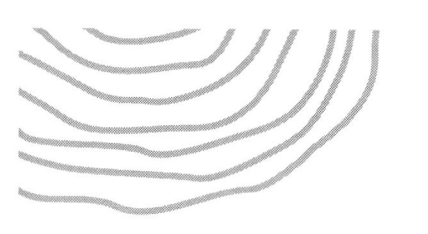

DATE

DATE

DATE

DATE

"What cannot be said will be wept."
~ Sappho

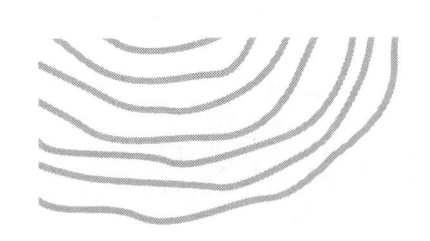

# Day 12

DATE

DATE

DATE

DATE

# Reflections

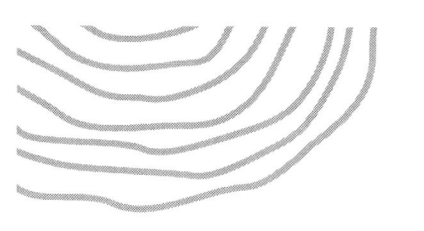

# Day 13

DATE

DATE

DATE

DATE

# Day 13

DATE

DATE

DATE

DATE

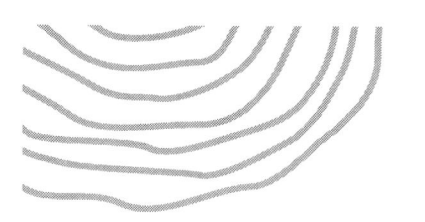

# Day 13

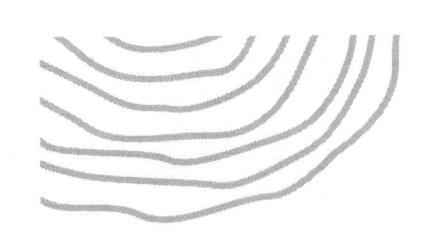

DATE

DATE

DATE

DATE

# Reflections

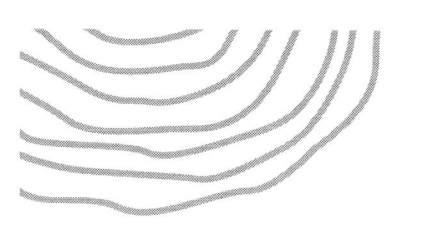

# Day 14

DATE

DATE

DATE

DATE

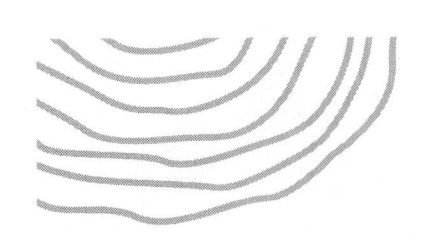

# Day 14

DATE

DATE

DATE

DATE

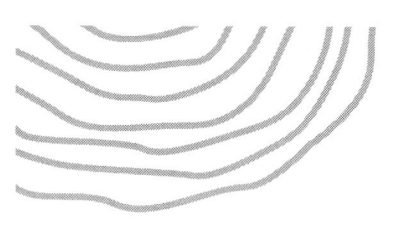

"The world is full of magic things, patiently waiting for our senses to grow sharper."
~ W. B. Yeats

# Day 14

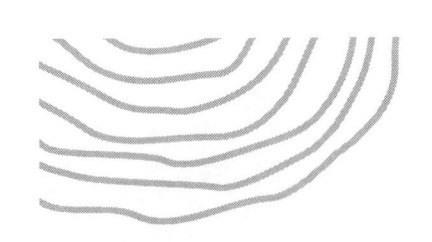

DATE

DATE

DATE

DATE

# Reflections

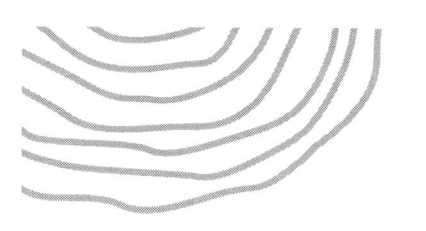

# Day 15

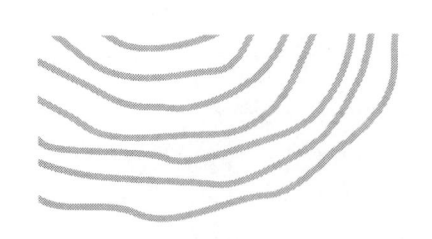

| DATE | | DATE | |
|---|---|---|---|

| DATE | | DATE | |
|---|---|---|---|

# Day 15

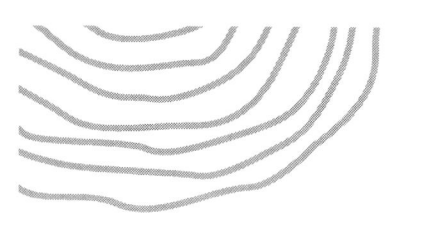

| DATE | | DATE | |
|------|--|------|--|

| DATE | | DATE | |
|------|--|------|--|

"We are all like the bright moon, we still have our darker side."
~ Kahil Gilbran

# Day 15

DATE

DATE

DATE

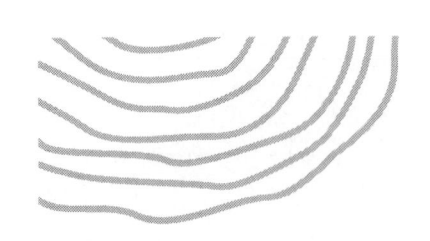

DATE

# Reflections

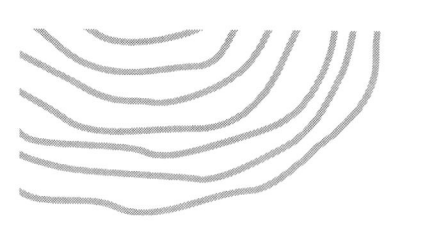

# Day 16

DATE

DATE

DATE

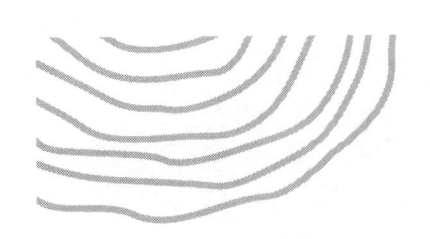

DATE

# Day 16

DATE

DATE

DATE

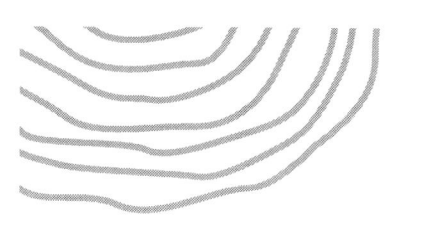

DATE

Always hold on to hope. Forget about the how

# Day 16

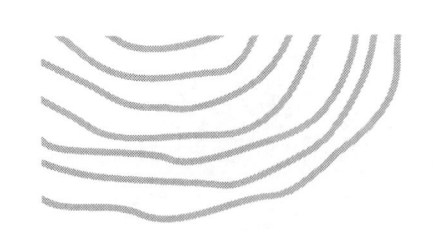

DATE

DATE

DATE

DATE

# Reflections

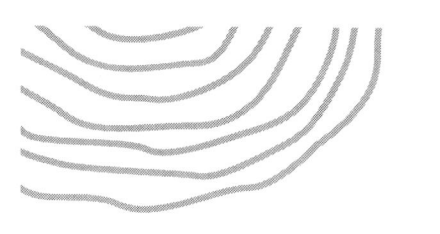

"Ah, what happiness it is to be with people who are all happy,
to press hands, press cheeks, smile into eyes."
~ Katherine Mansfield

# Day 17

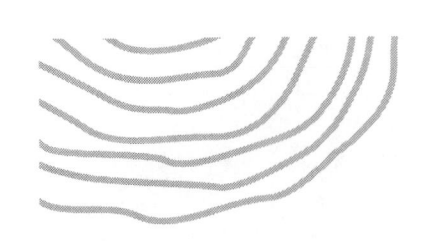

DATE

DATE

DATE

DATE

# Day 17

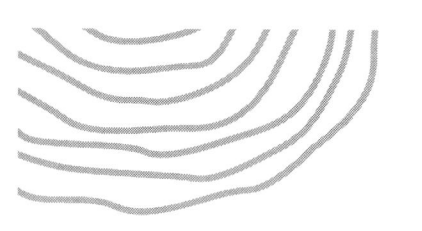

**DATE**

**DATE**

**DATE**

**DATE**

# Day 17

DATE

DATE

DATE

DATE

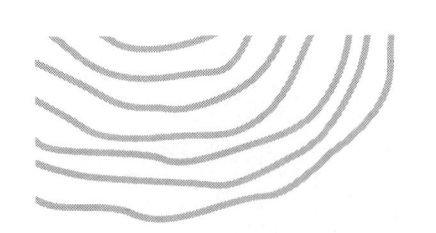

Choose joy

# Reflections

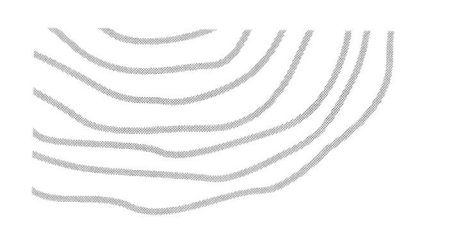

# Day 18

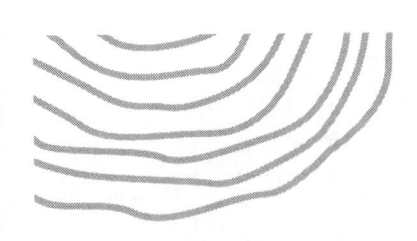

**DATE**

**DATE**

**DATE**

**DATE**

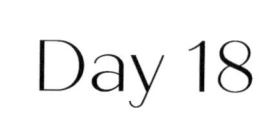

# Day 18

DATE

DATE

DATE

DATE

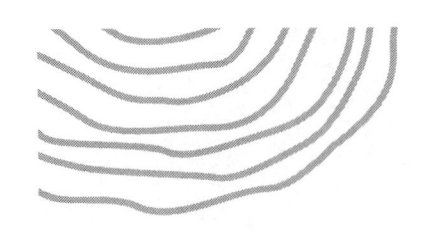

# Day 18

DATE

DATE

DATE

DATE

Keep it simple

# Reflections

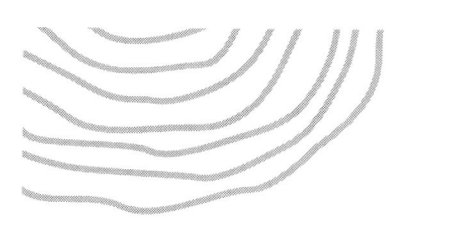

# Day 19

**DATE**

**DATE**

**DATE**

**DATE**

# Day 19

| DATE | DATE |
|---|---|

| DATE | DATE |

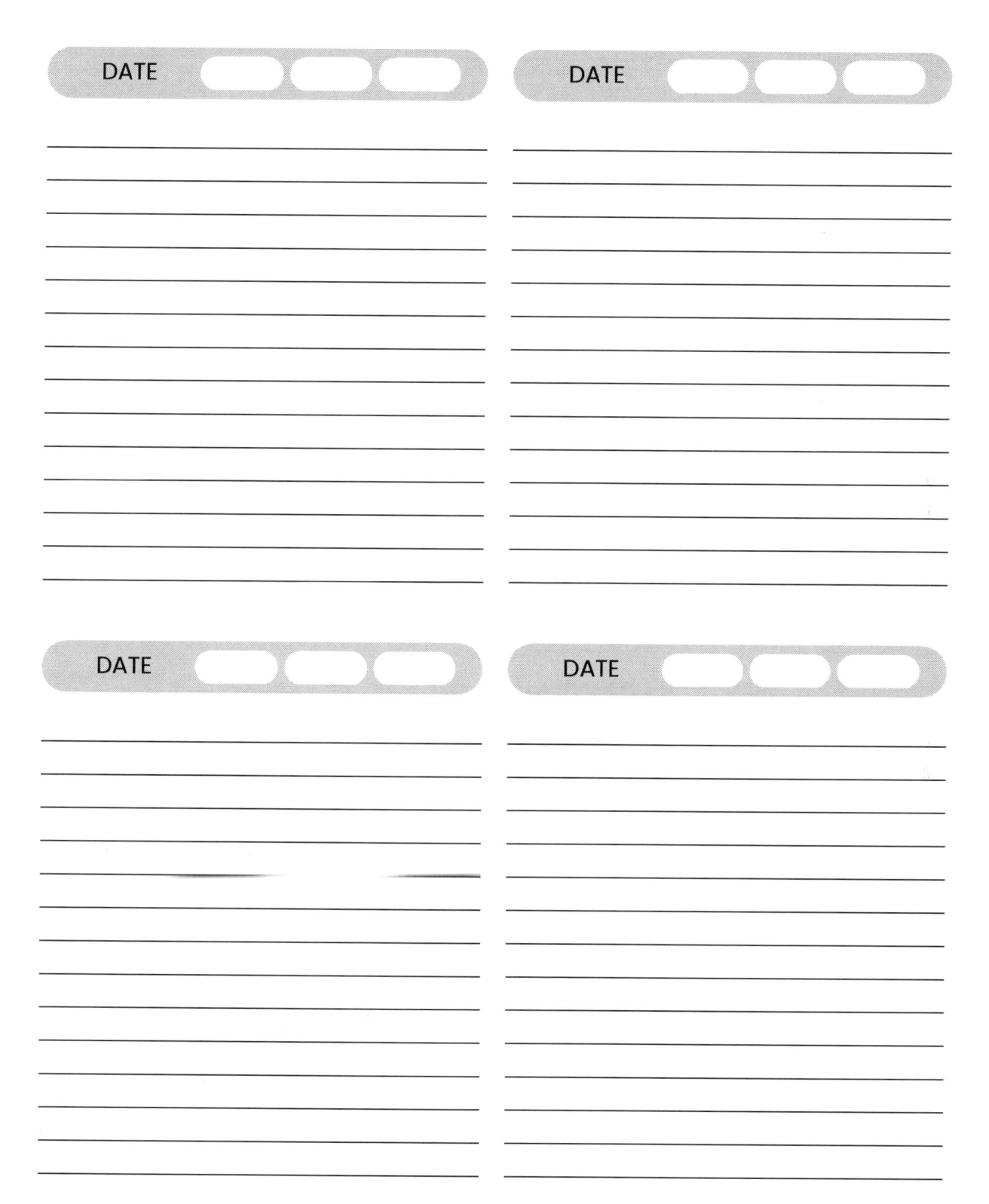

"Trust shows the way."
~ Hildegard von Bingen

# Day 19

DATE

DATE

DATE

DATE

# Reflections

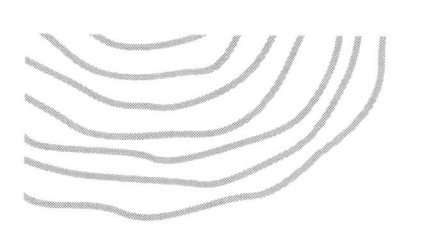

# Day 20

DATE

DATE

DATE

DATE

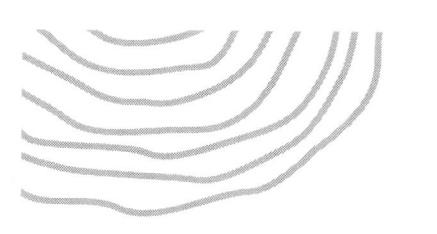

# Day 20

**DATE**

**DATE**

**DATE**

**DATE**

# Day 20

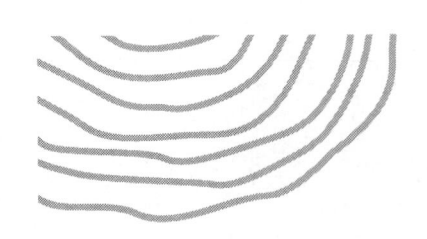

**DATE**

**DATE**

**DATE**

**DATE**

# Reflections

# Day 21

**DATE**

**DATE**

**DATE**

**DATE**

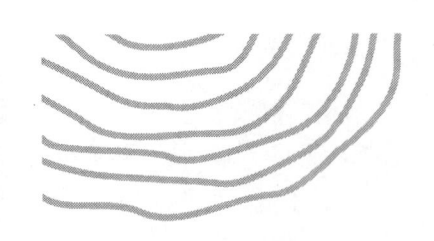

# Day 21

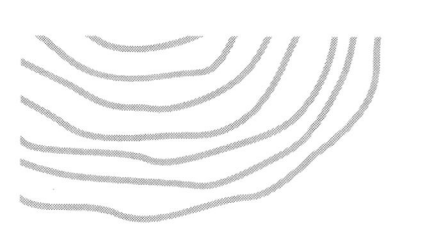

| DATE | | DATE | |

# Day 21

DATE

DATE

DATE

DATE

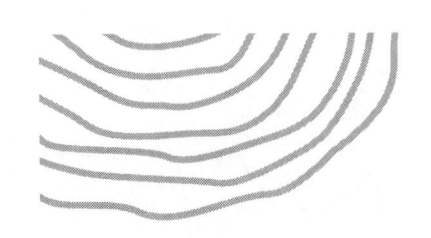

Easy does it

# Reflections

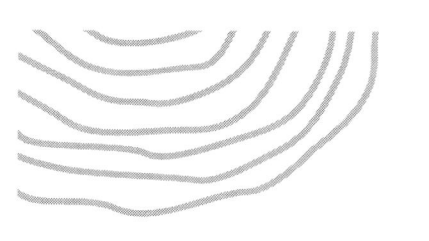

# Day 22

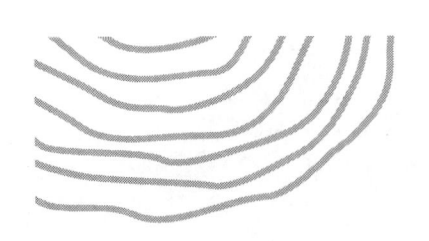

DATE

DATE

DATE

DATE

# Day 22

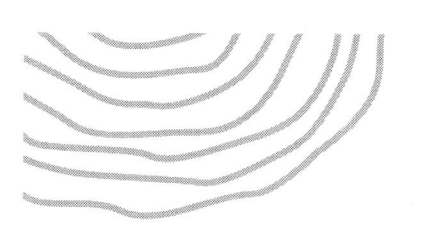

**DATE**

**DATE**

**DATE**

**DATE**

# Day 22

**DATE**

**DATE**

**DATE**

**DATE**

# Reflections

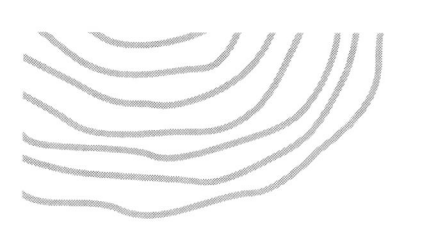

# Day 23

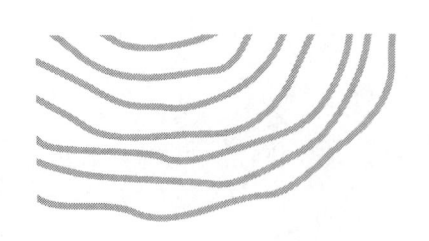

**DATE**

**DATE**

**DATE**

**DATE**

# Day 23

DATE

DATE

DATE

DATE

"After great pain, a formal feeling comes –The Nerves sit ceremonious, like Tombs"
~ Emily Dickinson

# Day 23

DATE

DATE

DATE

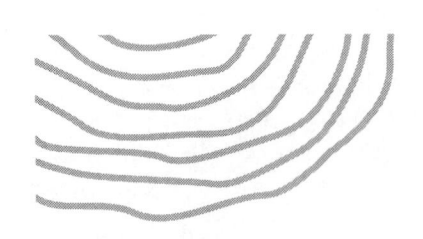

DATE

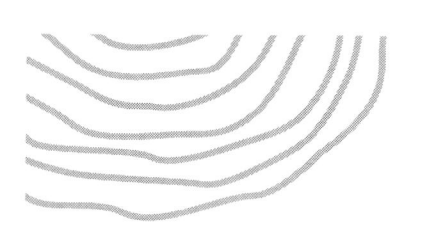

# Reflections

# Day 24

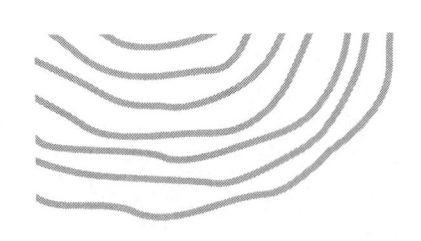

**DATE**

**DATE**

**DATE**

**DATE**

# Day 24

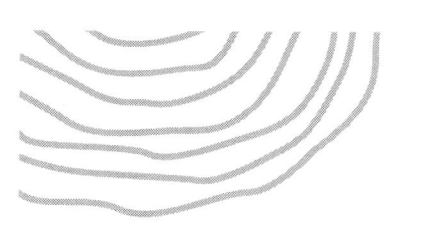

DATE

DATE

DATE

DATE

# Day 24

DATE

DATE

DATE

DATE

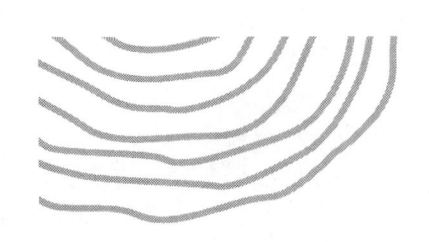

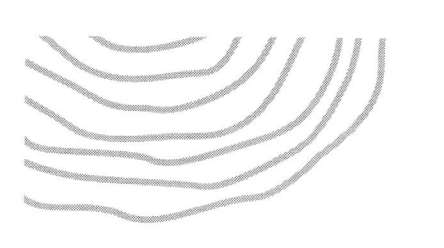

# Reflections

# Day 25

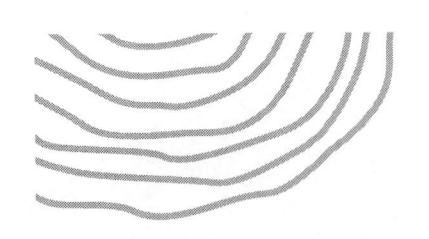

| DATE | | DATE | |
|---|---|---|---|

"It is almost as important to know what is not serious as to know what is"
~ John Kenneth Galbraith

# Day 25

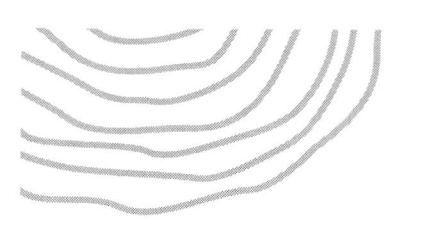

DATE

DATE

DATE

DATE

"When all else fails, write what your heart tells you"
~ Mark Twain

# Day 25

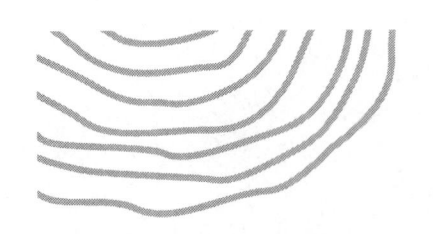

DATE

DATE

DATE

DATE

"Walking with a friend in the dark is better than walking alone in the light."
~ Helen Keller

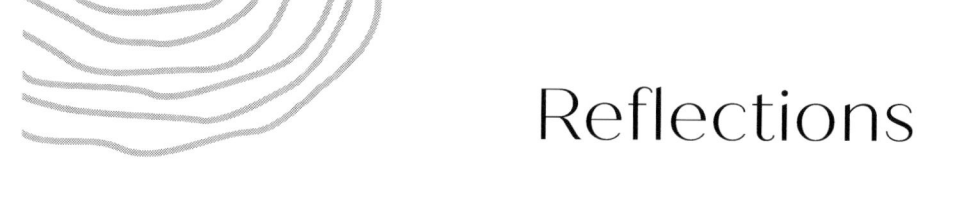

# Reflections

# Day 26

**DATE**

**DATE**

**DATE**

**DATE**

# Day 26

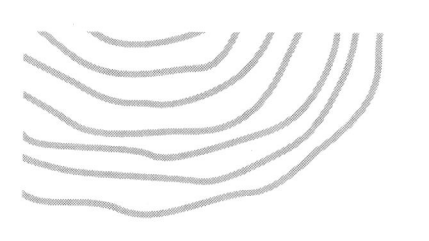

| DATE | DATE |
|---|---|
| DATE | DATE |

# Day 26

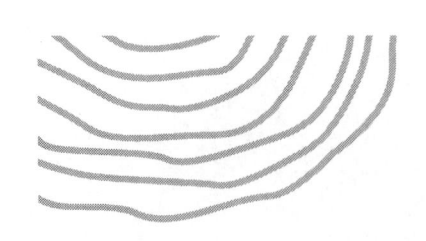

**DATE**

**DATE**

**DATE**

**DATE**

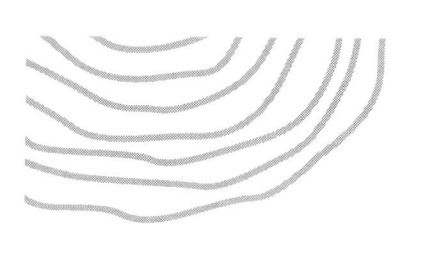

# Reflections

# Day 27

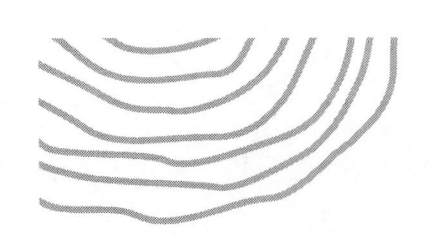

| DATE | | DATE | |
|---|---|---|---|

| DATE | | DATE | |
|---|---|---|---|

# Day 27

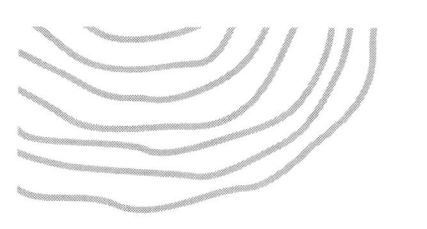

DATE

DATE

DATE

DATE

"Who has seen the wind? Neither you nor I but when the trees bow down their heads, the wind is passing by." ~ Christina Rossetti

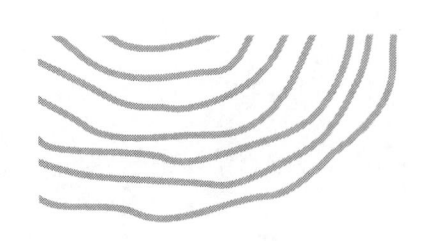

# Day 27

**DATE**

**DATE**

**DATE**

**DATE**

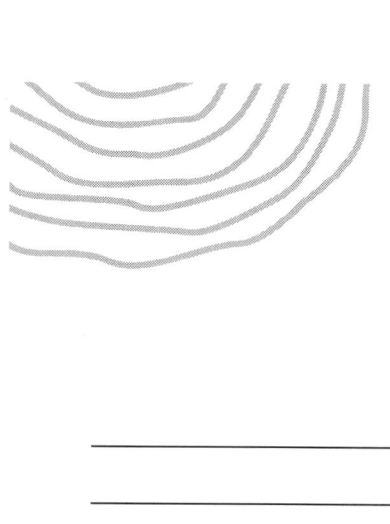

# Reflections

# Day 28

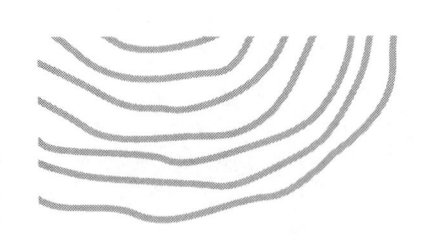

**DATE**

**DATE**

**DATE**

**DATE**

# Day 28

**DATE**

**DATE**

**DATE**

**DATE**

"None of us want to be in calm waters all our lives."
~ Jane Austen

# Day 28

**DATE**

**DATE**

**DATE**

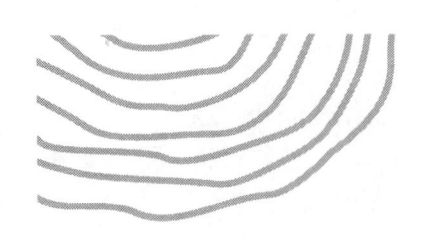

**DATE**

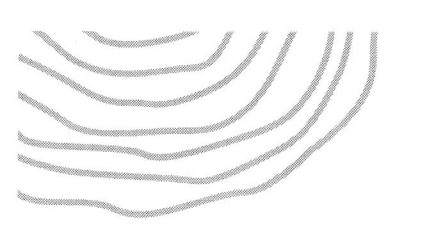

# Reflections

# Day 29

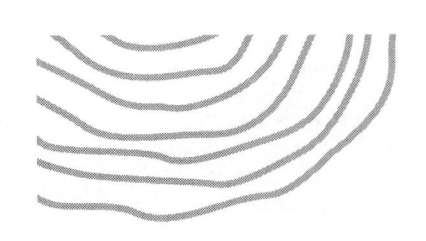

**DATE**

**DATE**

**DATE**

**DATE**

# Day 29

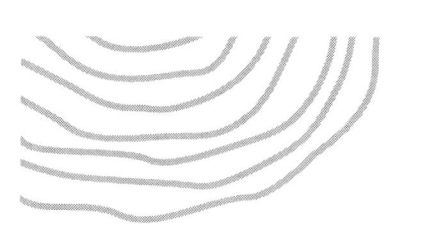

| DATE | DATE |
|---|---|

| DATE | DATE |

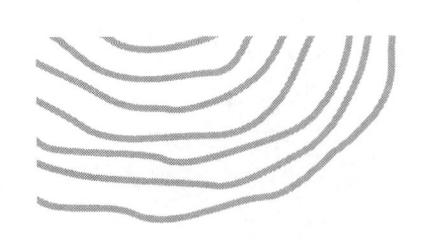

# Day 29

DATE

DATE

DATE

DATE

# Reflections

# Day 30

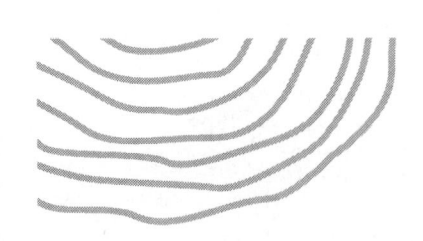

**DATE**

**DATE**

**DATE**

**DATE**

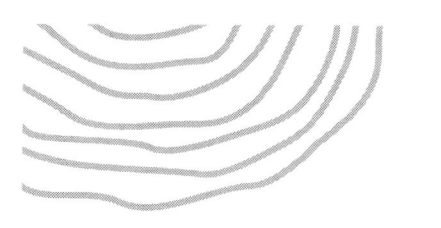

# Day 30

DATE

DATE

DATE

DATE

"If we take care of the moments, the years will take care of themselves."
~ Maria Edgeworth

# Day 30

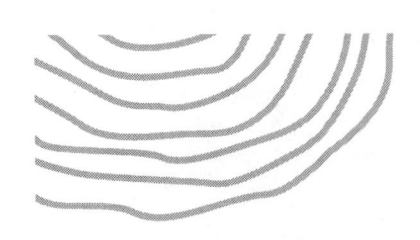

**DATE**

**DATE**

**DATE**

**DATE**

# Reflections

# Day 31

**DATE**

**DATE**

**DATE**

**DATE**

# Day 31

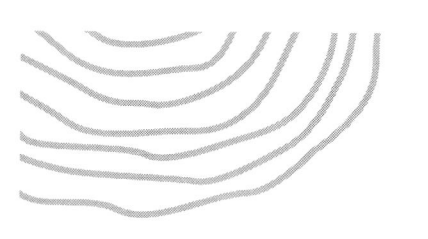

DATE

DATE

DATE

DATE

# Day 31

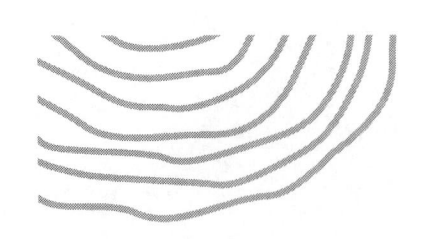

**DATE**

**DATE**

**DATE**

**DATE**

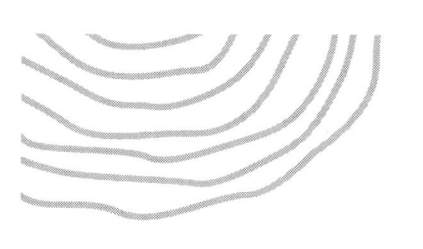

# Reflections

# Day 32

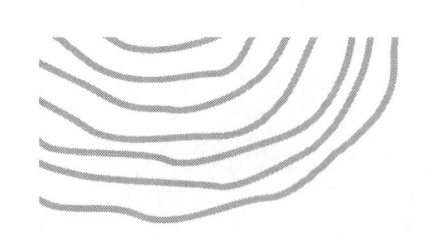

DATE

DATE

DATE

DATE

# Day 32

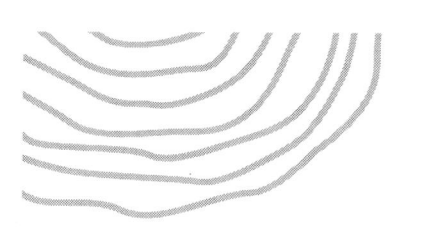

DATE

DATE

DATE

DATE

# Day 32

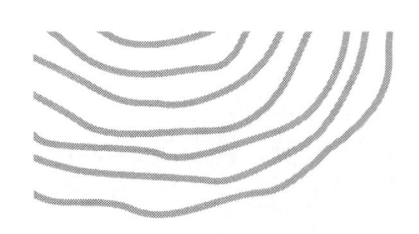

**DATE**

**DATE**

**DATE**

**DATE**

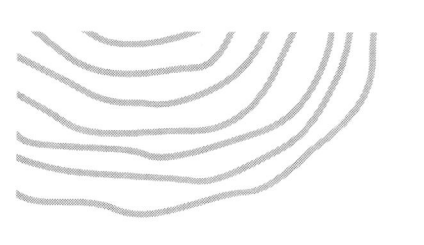

# Reflections

# Day 33

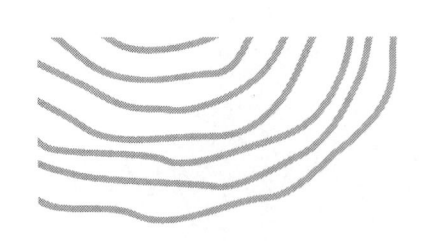

DATE

DATE

DATE

DATE

# Day 33

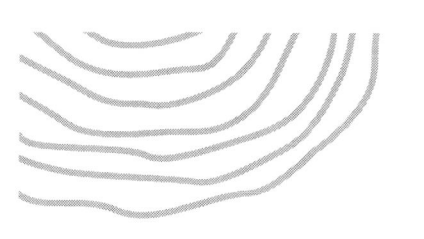

DATE

DATE

DATE

DATE

# Day 33

**DATE**

**DATE**

**DATE**

**DATE**

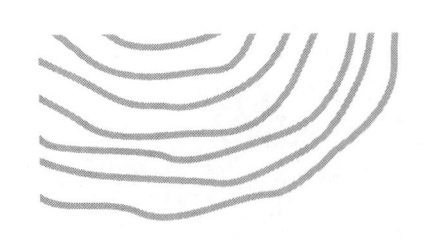

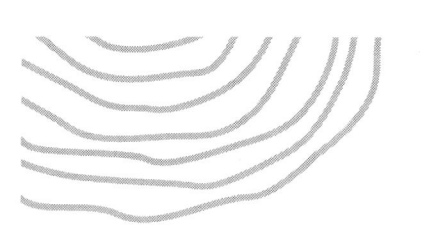

# Reflections

# Day 34

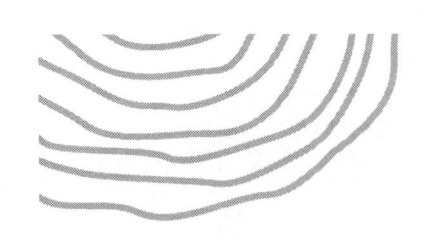

| DATE | | DATE | |
|---|---|---|---|

# Day 34

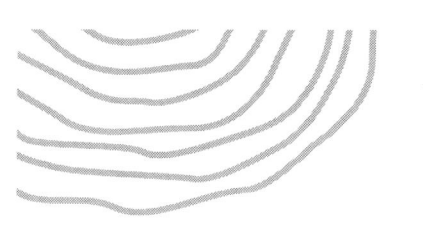

| DATE | | DATE | |
|---|---|---|---|

| DATE | | DATE | |
|---|---|---|---|

# Day 34

**DATE**

**DATE**

**DATE**

**DATE**

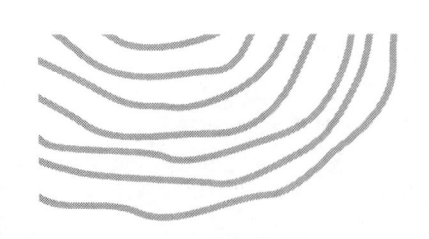

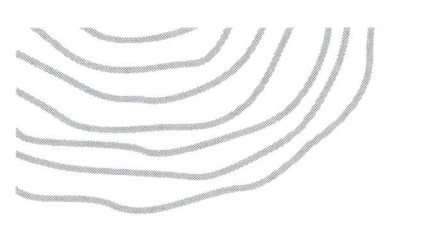

# Reflections

"If you bring forth that which is within you, then that which is within you will be your salvation. If you do not bring forth that which is within you, then that which is within you will destroy you."
~ The book of Thomas, The Bible

# Day 35

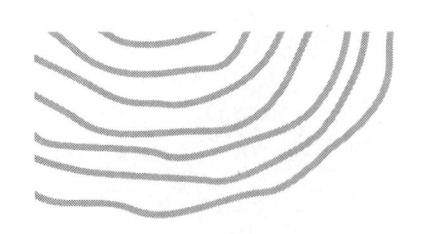

**DATE**

**DATE**

**DATE**

**DATE**

# Day 35

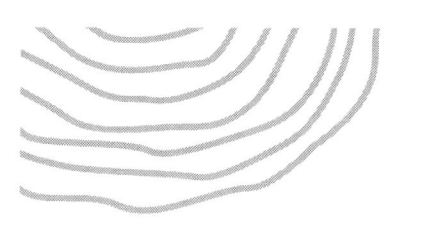

**DATE**

**DATE**

**DATE**

**DATE**

# Day 35

DATE

DATE

DATE

DATE

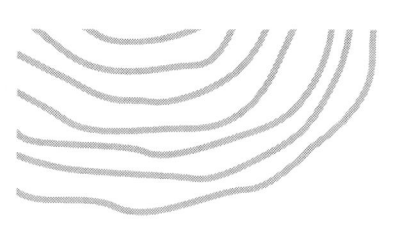

# Reflections

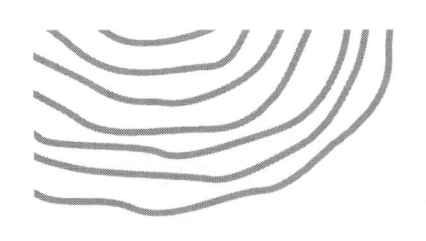

# About the author

**Lisa de Jong** is a womens' health coach specialising in the menstrual cycle, chronic pain, and trauma. Coming from years of debilitating period pain herself, she embarked on a journey of healing and self-discovery through the changing energies of the menstrual cycle. She has trained in various disciplines to support this work allowing for a mind-body-spirit approach.

Lisa offers 1:1 online coaching to clients all over the world, as well as talks and workshops to companies.

She is also the founder and facilitator of the globally accredited "Menstrual Cycle Coaching and Facilitation Professional Training" programme. This professional training is for anyone who would like to become a menstrual cycle coach or anyone looking to train in this field to support their existing professional practice or career.

Lisa hosts a podcast called "From Pain To Power," which you can find on all podcast platforms.

Find out more at www.lisadejongcoaching.com or Lisa's Instagram @lisa_dejong_coach

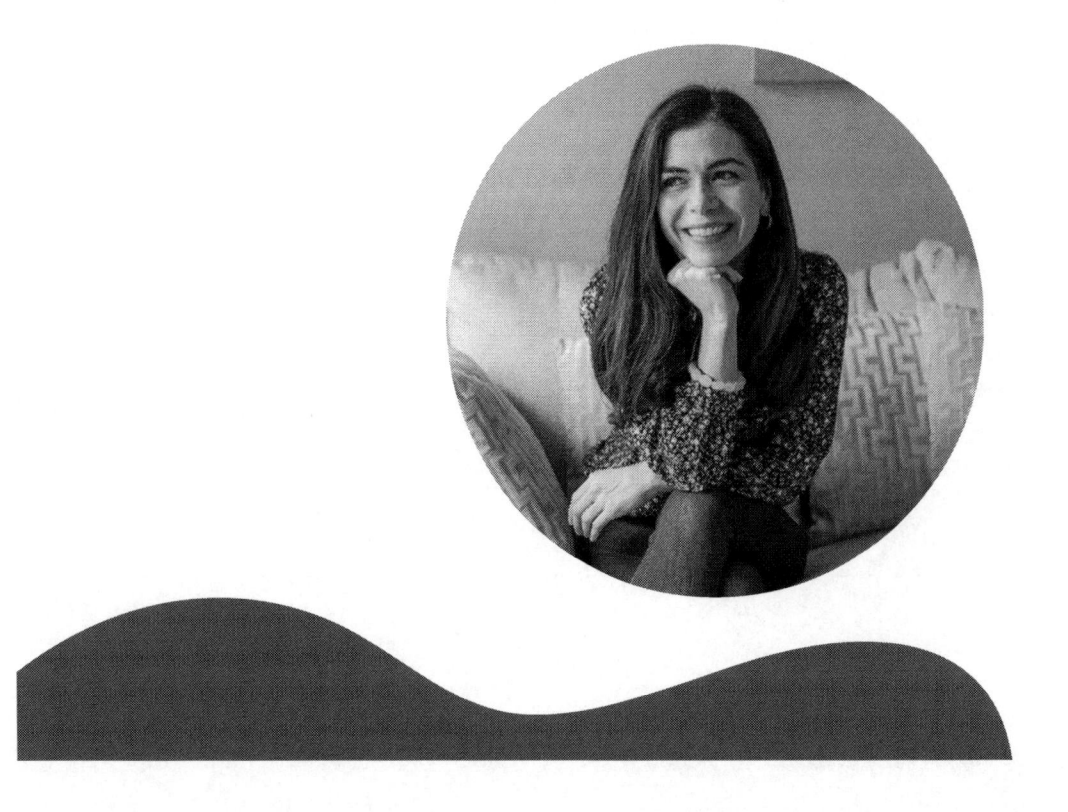

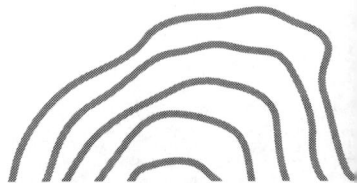

Printed in Great Britain
by Amazon